Anti- Inflammatory Diet For Beginners ;

A Guide to Enjoying Meals that Support Your Immune System Without Stress.

Nicole P. Wimer

Copyright Page

Disclaimer Page

The information provided in this cookbook by Carmen L. Perry is for educational and informational purposes only. It is not intended as medical advice, diagnosis, or treatment. Always consult with a qualified healthcare professional or nutritionist before making changes to your diet, especially if you have existing health conditions or concerns.

The recipes and dietary suggestions in this cookbook are based on general principles of anti-inflammatory eating. Individual nutritional needs may vary, and what works well for one person may not be suitable for another.

Carmen L. Perry and the publisher make no representations or warranties with respect to the accuracy, applicability, fitness, or completeness of the contents of this cookbook. They disclaim any warranties (expressed or implied), merchantability, or fitness for any particular purpose. Carmen L. Perry and the publisher shall have neither liability nor responsibility to any person or entity with respect to any loss, damage, or injury caused or alleged to be caused directly or indirectly by the information contained in this cookbook.

By using this cookbook, you agree to indemnify, defend, and hold harmless Carmen L. Perry and the publisher from any claims, losses, or damages resulting from your use or misuse of the information provided herein.

Eat responsibly, listen to your body, and enjoy nourishing, delicious meals on your journey to better health.

Author's Page

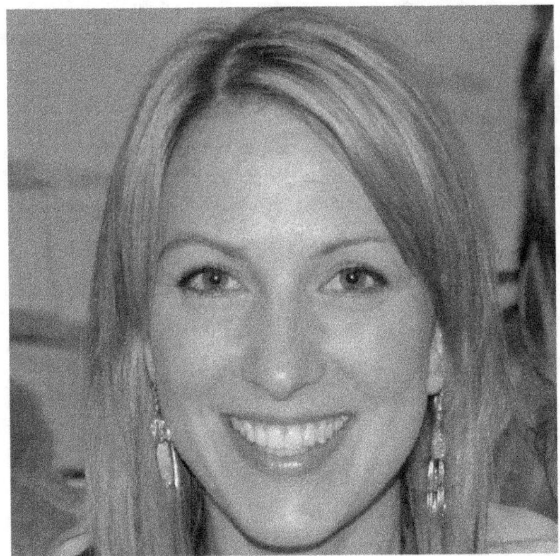

Nicole P. Wimmer is deeply committed to the field of nutrition, driven by her passion for holistic well-being and the promotion of healthy lifestyles. Over the years, she has amassed a wealth of expertise in nutritional science, consistently emphasizing the significance of balanced eating for enhancing overall health. Beyond her academic pursuits, Nicole genuinely believes in the profound healing capabilities of food, recognizing its ability to revitalize both the body and the spirit.

Witnessing the impactful effects of dietary choices on people's health firsthand, Nicole felt compelled to embark on a transformative mission. Her goal has been to educate, inspire, and empower individuals to make informed nutritional decisions. Through a combination of rigorous research, personalized consultations, and engaging community outreach initiatives, she has made a lasting impact on numerous lives, guiding them towards choices that align with their distinct nutritional requirements.

Nicole's approach to nutrition is far from one-size-fits-all; she artfully combines evidence-based practices with a compassionate touch. This ensures that every individual she works with receives advice tailored specifically to their unique circumstances and needs. Her wealth of knowledge, combined with her warm and empathetic demeanor, cultivates an environment of trust and understanding. As a result, her clients feel confident and enthusiastic about embarking on their personal wellness journeys.

In her cookbook, Nicole P. Wimmer channels her extensive experience and expertise into crafting recipes that do more than just satisfy taste buds. She designs dishes that nourish the body from the inside out, reflecting her genuine dedication to people's well-being. Each page of her cookbook emanates her heartfelt commitment to enhancing lives through the transformative power of anti-inflammatory eating.

Outside of her professional endeavors, Nicole enjoys exploring local farmers' markets, experimenting with innovative recipes in her own kitchen, and cherishing quality moments with her loved ones. Her holistic approach to life, both personally and professionally, stands as a testament to her enduring commitment to fostering health, happiness, and harmony for everyone she encounters.

Chapter 1: Introduction

Welcome to "Simple Healing: A Stress-Free Meal Guide for Boosting Your Immune System" by Carmen L. Perry. In the bustling world of modern nutrition, where fad diets come and go, the importance of an anti-inflammatory approach to eating remains steadfast. This cookbook is your gateway to understanding, embracing, and reaping the myriad benefits of an anti-inflammatory lifestyle.

Understanding Inflammation:

At its core, inflammation is the body's natural response to injury or infection, signaling the immune system to initiate healing. However, chronic inflammation—often triggered by factors like stress, poor diet, and environmental toxins—can lead to a host of health issues, including cardiovascular diseases, diabetes, arthritis, and more. Recognizing the distinction between acute and chronic inflammation is paramount, as it paves the way for informed dietary choices.

Benefits of an Anti-Inflammatory Diet:
Adopting an anti-inflammatory diet isn't merely a fleeting trend; it's a conscious decision to prioritize your health and well-being. By incorporating foods rich in antioxidants, omega-3 fatty acids, and phytonutrients, you can mitigate inflammation, enhance immune function, improve digestion, and bolster overall vitality. From heightened energy levels to improved cognitive function and radiant skin, the benefits are both profound and far-reaching.

Key Nutrients and Foods that Fight Inflammation:

Navigating the vast landscape of anti-inflammatory foods can seem daunting, but fear not! This cookbook demystifies the process, spotlighting key nutrients and ingredients that are your allies in the fight against inflammation. From vibrant berries bursting with antioxidants to omega-3-packed fish like salmon, and from the golden hues of turmeric to the wholesome goodness of leafy greens and nuts—each recipe is a testament to nature's bounty and its unparalleled healing potential.

Tips for Transitioning to an Anti-Inflammatory Lifestyle:
Embarking on an anti-inflammatory journey is a transformative experience—one that requires patience, commitment, and a sprinkle of culinary creativity. Whether you're a seasoned health enthusiast or taking your first steps toward wellness, this cookbook offers invaluable tips, strategies, and insights to guide your transition seamlessly. From mindful meal planning and savvy grocery shopping to cultivating a supportive environment and nurturing self-care practices, Carmen L. Perry's expertise shines through, empowering you to embrace this nourishing lifestyle with confidence and joy.

In essence, "Simple Healing" is more than just a cookbook; it's a companion, a guide, and a beacon of hope for anyone seeking to harness the transformative power of anti-inflammatory eating. With Carmen's compassionate guidance and delectable recipes at your fingertips, you're poised to embark on a journey that transcends the confines of mere nutrition—it's a journey toward holistic health, radiant vitality, and a life brimming with abundance.

10 Benefits of Following "Simple Healing" Cookbook:

- Enhanced Well-being: Adopting an anti-inflammatory diet can promote overall health, leading to increased energy levels and vitality.
- Reduced Inflammation: By incorporating anti-inflammatory foods and recipes, you may experience a decrease in chronic inflammation, potentially alleviating associated symptoms.
- Improved Digestion: Many recipes in this cookbook are designed to support gut health, aiding in better digestion and nutrient absorption.
- Weight Management: A balanced anti-inflammatory diet can assist in weight regulation by promoting satiety and supporting metabolic health.

- Enhanced Immune Function: By nourishing your body with immune-boosting nutrients, you can bolster your natural defenses against illnesses and infections.
- Radiant Skin: Nutrient-dense ingredients in these recipes can contribute to healthier skin, reducing inflammation-related skin conditions.
- Mental Clarity: Consuming foods rich in omega-3 fatty acids and antioxidants may support brain health, enhancing cognitive function and mood.
- Heart Health: Many ingredients in this cookbook, such as fatty fish and nuts, are beneficial for cardiovascular health, supporting optimal heart function.
- Versatile Recipes: "Simple Healing" offers a diverse range of recipes, ensuring that you can enjoy flavorful meals while adhering to an anti-inflammatory lifestyle.
- Empowerment: By equipping yourself with knowledge and practical recipes, you gain the tools to take control of your health and well-being, fostering a sense of empowerment and autonomy.

10 Encouragements for Beginners:

- Start Slowly: Embrace gradual changes, incorporating one or two new recipes each week to ease into the anti-inflammatory lifestyle.
- Celebrate Small Wins: Recognize and celebrate your progress, no matter how minor it may seem. Every step forward is a victory.
- Stand by listening to Your Body: Focus on how various food sources cause you to feel, and change your eating regimen appropriately. Your body is your best guide.
- Seek Support: Connect with like-minded individuals, join online communities, or seek guidance from healthcare professionals to stay motivated and informed.
- Experiment and Explore: Embrace culinary exploration, trying new ingredients and flavor combinations to keep your meals exciting and satisfying.
- Plan Ahead: Invest time in meal planning and preparation to set yourself up for success. Batch cooking and meal prepping can be invaluable tools.
- Stay Hydrated: Drink plenty of water and herbal teas to support detoxification and overall hydration, essential for optimal health.
- Practice Mindfulness: Cultivate mindfulness during meals, savoring each bite, and appreciating the nourishment you're providing your body.
- Embrace Adaptability: Recollect that flawlessness isn't the objective.Allow yourself grace and flexibility, acknowledging that occasional indulgences are part of a balanced lifestyle.

- Stay Inspired: Keep the momentum going by exploring new recipes, reading inspiring health-related literature, and reminding yourself of the profound benefits of your anti-inflammatory journey.
- Setting out on another dietary excursion can be both energizing and testing, yet with devotion, support, and a sprinkle of innovativeness, you're exceptional to embrace the groundbreaking force of "Basic Recovering" and embarked on a path to incredible success and fortune.

Chapter 2: Breakfast Delights

1. Spinach & Egg Scramble With Raspberries

Prep Time:10 mins
Total Time:10 mins
Servings:1
Yield:1 serving

Ingredients

1. 1 teaspoon canola oil
2. 1 ½ cups child spinach (1 1/2 ounces)
3. 2 huge eggs, delicately beaten
4. Touch of legitimate salt
5. Touch of ground pepper
6. 1 cut entire grain bread, toasted
7. ½ cup new raspberries

Bearings

Heat oil in a little nonstick skillet over medium-high intensity. Add spinach and cook until withered, mixing frequently, 1 to 2 minutes. Move the spinach to a plate.

Clean the container off, place over medium intensity and add eggs. Cook, blending on more than one occasion to guarantee in any event, cooking, until recently set, 1 to 2 minutes. Mix in the spinach, salt and pepper. Present the scramble with raspberries and bread.

2. Southwest Waffle

Prep Time:10 mins
Total Time:10 mins
Servings:1
Yield:1 waffle

Ingredients

1. 1 frozen entire grain waffle, like Van's 8 Entire Grains Multigrain
2. 1 egg, concocted bright side
3. ¼ medium avocado, split, cultivated, stripped and slashed
4. 1 tablespoon refrigerated new salsa

Bearings

Toast waffle as per bundle headings. Top with egg, avocado, and salsa.

3. Egg Salad Avocado Toast

Prep Time:5 mins
Total Time:5 mins
Servings:1
Yield:1 toast

Ingredients

1. ¼ avocado
2. 1 tablespoon celery
3. ½ teaspoon lemon juice
4. ½ teaspoon hot sauce
5. Spot of salt
6. 1 cleaved hard-bubbled egg
7. 1 cut entire wheat toast

Bearings

Squash avocado with celery, lemon juice, hot sauce and salt in a little bowl. Blend in a hard-bubbled egg. Spread on toast.

4. Smoked Salmon & Cream Cheese Omelet

Cook Time:15 mins
Total Time:15 mins
Servings:1
Yield:1 serving

Ingredients

1. 2 huge eggs
2. 1 teaspoon decreased fat milk or water
3. ⅛ teaspoon ground pepper, in addition to something else for decorate
4. Touch of salt
5. 1 teaspoon spread
6. 2 tablespoons hacked smoked salmon
7. 1 tablespoon cream cheddar, mellowed, or disintegrated feta
8. 1 tablespoon finely hacked red onion
9. 1 ½ teaspoons hacked new dill, in addition to something else for decorate

Headings

Whisk eggs, milk (or water), pepper and salt in a little bowl.

Soften spread in a little nonstick skillet over medium-low intensity, shifting the dish to ensure the whole base is covered. Add the egg combination and cook for 1 moment without blending. Sprinkle salmon, cheddar, onion and dill more than one portion of the eggs. Cook for 1 moment. Utilizing an adaptable spatula, lift the uncovered side to let crude egg from the center stream under; you might have to marginally shift the dish. Keep lifting in various spots until there's basically no crude egg on top. Cook for 2 minutes more.

Utilizing the spatula, flip the exposed side over the filling, collapsing the omelet down the middle, and cook for 1 moment. (Assuming the eggs are beginning to brown, bring down the intensity.) Cautiously flip the omelet over and cook brief more. Serve right away, embellished with more dill and pepper, whenever wanted.

5. Breakfast Salad With Eggs & Salsa Verde Vinaigrette

Prep Time:10 mins
Total Time:10 mins
Servings:1
Yield:1 serving

Ingredients

1. 2 large eggs
2. 1 teaspoon reduced-fat milk or water
3. 1/2 tsp ground pepper, plus additional for decoration
4. A dash of salt
5. One tsp of butter
6. Chop two teaspoons of smoked salmon
7. One tablespoon of softened feta cheese or crumbled cream cheese
8. One tablespoon of red onion, diced finely
9. One-third cup finely chopped fresh dill, plus extra for decoration

Directions

Whisk eggs, milk (or water), pepper and salt in a small bowl.

In a small nonstick skillet over medium-low heat, melt butter, turning the pan to cover the entire bottom. Stir in the egg mixture and simmer, stirring, for one minute. Over one half of the eggs, scatter the salmon, cheese, onion, and dill. Simmer for one minute. Lift the exposed side with a flexible spatula to allow the raw egg from the center to trickle underneath; the pan might need to be gently tipped. Lift in various places until nearly no raw egg remains on top. Cook for an additional two minutes.

Fold the omelet in half, flip the bare side over the filling with the spatula, and cook for one minute. (If the eggs are starting to brown, lower the heat.) Carefully flip the omelet over and cook 1 minute more. Serve immediately, garnished with more dill and pepper, if desired.

6. Cherry Mocha Smoothie

Prep Time:10 mins
Total Time:10 mins
Servings:2
Yield:2 servings

Ingredients

1 cup frozen unsweetened pitted dim sweet cherries
1 cup unsweetened chocolate almond milk
5.3 to 6-ounce container vanilla sans fat Greek yogurt
½ medium banana (see Tip)
2 tablespoons unsweetened cocoa powder
2 tablespoons almond margarine
1 teaspoon moment coffee espresso powder
1 teaspoon vanilla
2 cups ice shapes
1 tablespoon Dim chocolate shavings, chocolate-covered coffee beans

Headings

In a blender join the cherries, almond milk, Greek yogurt, banana, cocoa powder, almond margarine, coffee espresso powder and vanilla. Cover and mix until smooth. Add ice shapes; cover and mix until smooth. Fill glasses and whenever wanted, top with chocolate shavings, chocolate-covered coffee beans or potentially extra banana cuts (see Tip).

Tips

Tips: Strip remaining banana half, wrap firmly in saran wrap, then, at that point, in foil. Freeze for a sometime in the future.
Assuming you like, partition the ice 3D shapes between two tall glasses as opposed to mixing the ice with the smoothie. To serve, pour smoothie over the ice solid shapes.
Variety: This recipe effectively pairs to make four servings. Make the full recipe on the double, then fill bricklayer containers with tight fitting covers. Store in the cooler. The prior night serving, move container to the refrigerator to defrost.

7. **Mango- Almond Smoothie Bowl**

Prep Time:10 mins
Total Time:10 mins
Servings:1
Yield:1 serving

Ingredients

1. ½ cup frozen hacked mango
2. ½ cup nonfat plain Greek yogurt
3. ¼ cup frozen cut banana
4. ¼ cup plain unsweetened almond milk
5. 5 tablespoons unsalted almonds, separated
6. ⅛ teaspoon ground allspice
7. ¼ cup raspberries
8. ½ teaspoon honey

Bearings

Mix mango, yogurt, banana, almond milk, 3 tablespoons of almonds and allspice in a blender until exceptionally smooth.

Empty the smoothie into a bowl and top with raspberries, the leftover 2 tablespoons of almonds and honey.

8. **Beans On Toast**

Active Time:
20 mins
Total Time:
20 mins
Servings:
4

Ingredients
1. 1 tablespoon unsalted margarine
2. 3 cups meagerly cut cremini mushrooms
3. 1 ½ tablespoons lower-sodium Worcestershire sauce
4. 2 teaspoons tomato glue
5. ¾ teaspoon bean stew powder
6. ¼ teaspoon salt
7. 1 (13.7-ounce) can heated beans in pureed tomatoes (like Heinz)
8. 4 cuts multigrain bread, toasted
9. 1 tablespoon slashed new level leaf parsley

Headings
Soften margarine in a huge pan over medium-high intensity. Add mushrooms; cook, blending at times, until they start to mellow, around 5 minutes.

Lessen intensity to medium; add Worcestershire, tomato glue, bean stew powder and salt; mix until all around consolidated. Cook, blending at times, until the fluid has dissipated and the mushrooms are brilliant brown, around 5 minutes.

Diminish intensity to low and add beans; cook, blending every so often, until completely warmed, 3 to 5 minutes.
Spoon 1/2 cup of the bean combination onto each cut of toast and sprinkle with parsley.

9. Egg Sandwiches With Rosemary, Tomato & Feta

Prep Time:5 mins
Additional Time:15 mins
Total Time:20 mins
Servings:4
Yield:4 servings

Ingredients
4 multigrain sandwich diminishes
4 teaspoons olive oil
1 tablespoon clipped new rosemary or 1/2 teaspoon dried rosemary, squashed
4 eggs
2 cups new child spinach leaves
1 medium tomato, cut into 8 slight cuts
4 tablespoons diminished fat feta cheddar
⅛ teaspoon legitimate salt
Newly ground dark pepper

Headings
Preheat broiler to 375°F. Part sandwich diminishes; brush cut sides with 2 teaspoons of the olive oil. Put on rimmed baking sheet; toast in stove around 5 minutes or until edges are light brown and fresh.

In the mean time, in an enormous skillet heat the excess 2 teaspoons olive oil and the rosemary over medium-high intensity. Break eggs, each in turn, into skillet. Cook around 1 moment or until whites are set yet yolks are as yet runny. Break yolks with spatula. Flip eggs; cook on the opposite side until done. Eliminate from heat.

Place the base parts of the toasted sandwich diminishes on 4 serving plates. Split spinach between sandwich diminishes on plates. Top each with 2 of the tomato cuts, an egg and 1 tablespoon of the feta cheddar. Sprinkle with the salt and pepper. Top with the excess sandwich meager parts.

10. **Sweet Potato , Corn & Black Beans Hash**

Cook Time:35 mins
Total Time:35 mins
Servings:2
Yield:2 servings, about cups each

Ingredients

1. 2 teaspoons canola oil
2. 2 medium onions, hacked
3. 1 medium yam, stripped and cut into 1/2-inch dice
4. 2 huge cloves garlic, minced
5. 1 jalapeño pepper, cultivated and minced
6. 4 teaspoons ground cumin
7. ½ teaspoon salt
8. ¾ cup water
9. ¾ cup frozen corn pieces
10. 1 15-ounce can dark beans, washed
11. 2 tablespoons cleaved new cilantro
12. Newly ground pepper, to taste
13. 1 lime, cut into wedges

Bearings

Heat oil in a huge cast-iron skillet over medium-high intensity. Add onions and saute until seared in spots, 3 to 5 minutes. Add yam and cook, mixing, until it begins to brown in spots, 5 to 7 minutes. Mix in garlic, jalapeno, cumin and salt; saute until fragrant, around 30 seconds.

Add water and cook, scraping up any sautéed bits, until fluid is retained, 3 to 5 minutes. Mix in corn and dark beans and cook until warmed through. Mix in cilantro and season with salt and pepper. Present with lime wedges.

11. **Spring Green Frittata**

Prep Time:25 mins
Total Time:25 mins
Servings:2
Yield:2 servings

Ingredients

1. 2 eggs, gently beaten
2. 4 egg whites
3. 2 tablespoons sans fat milk
4. 1 teaspoon cut new chives
5. ⅛ teaspoon dark pepper
6. ¼ cup finely destroyed Parmesan cheddar (1 ounce)
7. 2 teaspoons olive oil
8. ½ cup 1/2-inch pieces asparagus
9. ¼ cup cut green onions
10. ½ cup coarsely slashed spinach leaves
11. 1 clove garlic, minced
12. 1 little roma tomato, cleaved

Headings

Preheat the grill. In a little bowl join the eggs, egg whites, milk, chives and pepper: mix in 2 tablespoons of the cheddar.

In an 8-inch nonstick grill verification skillet heat oil done on both sides. Add asparagus and green onions; cook and mix for 2 minutes. Add spinach and garlic; cook for 30 seconds or just until spinach is shriveled.

Empty egg blend into skillet; lessen intensity to low.

Cook, covered, 10 to 12 minutes or until almost set.

Sprinkle with 2 tablespoons cheddar.

Place the skillet under the oven 4 to 5 crawls from heat. Sear 1 moment or just until the top is set and the cheddar is dissolved. Top with tomato.

Chapter 3: Lunchtime Favorites

1. Cucumber, Tomato & Arugula Salad With Hummus

Cook Time: 10 mins
Total Time: 10 mins
Servings: 1
Yield: 1 serving

Ingredients

2 cups arugula
⅓ cup cherry tomatoes, split
⅓ cup cut cucumber
1 tablespoon cleaved red onion
1 ½ tablespoons extra-virgin olive oil
2 teaspoons red-wine vinegar
⅛ teaspoon ground pepper
1 tablespoon feta cheddar
1 4-inch entire wheat pita
¼ cup hummus

Bearings

Throw arugula in a bowl with tomatoes, cucumber, onion, oil, vinegar and pepper. Top with feta. Present with pita and hummus.

2. Mashed Chickpeas Salad With Dill & Capers

Prep Time:10 mins
Total Time:10 mins
Servings:4
Yield:2 cups

Ingredients
1 (15 ounce) can low-sodium chickpeas, flushed
⅓ cup finely slashed celery
¼ cup vegetarian mayonnaise
¼ cup slashed new dill
1 scallion, finely slashed
2 teaspoons escapades, cleaved
2 teaspoons lemon juice or more to taste
¼ teaspoon ground pepper

Headings
Place chickpeas in a spotless kitchen towel. Crease the towel over and delicately rub the chickpeas to deliver any free skins. Dispose of the skins; move the chickpeas to a medium bowl. Squash the chickpeas with a fork. Add celery, mayonnaise, dill, scallion, tricks, lemon squeeze and pepper; mix until all around covered.

Tips
To make ahead: Cover and refrigerate for as long as 4 days.

3. Crispy Chickpeas Bowl With Lemon Vinaigrette

Prep Time:35 mins
Additional Time:10 mins
Total Time:45 mins
Servings:4
Yield:4 servings

Ingredients

1. ⅔ cup quinoa
2. 1 ⅓ cups water in addition to 1 tablespoon, separated
3. ⅛ teaspoon salt in addition to 1/4 teaspoon, separated
4. 1 (15 ounce) can no-salt-added chickpeas, washed
5. 1 little red onion, daintily cut
6. 4 teaspoons extra-virgin olive oil in addition to 2 tablespoons, separated
7. ¼ teaspoon ground pepper, separated
8. 1 pack kale, stems eliminated, daintily cut (around 5 cups)
9. 1 teaspoon Dijon mustard
10. 1 clove garlic, minced
11. 2 teaspoons lemon zing
12. 2 tablespoons lemon juice
13. 1 red chime pepper, meagerly cut
14. ¼ cup disintegrated feta cheddar
15. 2 tablespoons toasted pumpkin seeds

Bearings

Preheat the stove to 400 degrees F. Cover a huge rimmed baking sheet generously with a cooking shower.

Consolidate quinoa, 1 1/3 cups water, and 1/8 teaspoon salt in a medium pan. Heat to the point of boiling over medium-high intensity. Decrease intensity to medium-low, somewhat cover, and stew until the quinoa is delicate, around 15 minutes. Channel any overabundance of water.

In the interim, wipe chickpeas off with a paper towel. Throw with onion, 2 teaspoons oil, and 1/8 teaspoon each salt and pepper in a huge bowl. Spread out on the pre-arranged baking sheet. Cook for 15 minutes.

Throw kale with 2 teaspoons of oil and the excess 1/8 teaspoon salt in the huge bowl. Mix the kale into the chickpeas and dish for 15 minutes more.

Whisk mustard, garlic, lemon zing, lemon squeeze, the leftover 1 tablespoon water and the excess 1/8 teaspoon pepper in a little bowl. Race in the leftover 2 tablespoons of oil.

Partition the quinoa among 4 serving bowls. Top with the kale combination, chime pepper cuts, feta, and pumpkin seeds. Sprinkle with the vinaigrette.

4. **Sweet Potato & Cauliflower Rice Bowl**

Prep Time:40 mins
Total Time:40 mins
Servings:4
Yield:4 servings

Ingredients

1. 1 medium yam, stripped whenever wanted, cut 1/4 inch thick
2. 2 teaspoons extra-virgin olive oil in addition to 2 tablespoons, isolated
3. 2 squeezes salt in addition to 1/2 teaspoon, isolated
4. ½ teaspoon ground pepper, isolated
5. ¼ cup squeezed orange
6. 2 tablespoons lime juice
7. ½ cup slashed new cilantro, isolated
8. 3 cloves garlic, minced, isolated
9. ½ teaspoon ground cumin
10. ½ teaspoon dried oregano
11. 5 cups cauliflower florets
12. 1 (15 ounce) can dark beans, flushed
13. 1 firm ready avocado, cut
14. ½ cup pico de gallo

Headings

Preheat the broiler to 400 degrees F.

Throw yam in a medium bowl with 2 teaspoons of oil, a spot of salt and 1/4 teaspoon pepper. Move to a baking sheet. Cook until delicate, 10 to 14 minutes

In the meantime, consolidate squeezed orange, lime juice, 1/4 cup cilantro, 1 minced garlic clove, cumin, oregano and a touch of salt in a little bowl.

Beat cauliflower florets in two clusters in a food processor until slashed into rice-size pieces. Heat the leftover 2 tablespoons of oil in a huge skillet over medium intensity.

Add the leftover 2 garlic cloves and cook until fragrant, around 30 seconds. Add the cauliflower rice, the leftover 1/2 teaspoon salt and 1/4 teaspoon pepper; cook, blending, until relaxed, 3 to 5 minutes. Eliminate from intensity and mix in the leftover 1/4 cup cilantro.

To serve, split the cauliflower between 4 dishes. Top with the yam, dark beans, avocado and pico de gallo. Shower each piece with the magic sauce.

5. Black Bean Wraps With Green & Cilantro Vinaigrette

Active Time:20 mins
Total Time:20 mins
Servings:4

Ingredients

1. 1 cup cleaved new cilantro
2. 3 tablespoons white-wine vinegar
3. 2 cloves garlic, stripped
4. 1 teaspoon ground cumin, partitioned
5. ½ teaspoon salt, partitioned
6. ¼ cup extra-virgin olive oil
7. 3 cups cleaved romaine lettuce
8. 1 cup cleaved radicchio
9. 1 cup cut radishes
10. 1 (15 ounce) can no-salt-added dark beans, flushed
11. ½ teaspoon bean stew powder
12. ½ teaspoon garlic powder
13. 1 ready avocado
14. 1 tablespoon lime juice
15. 4 (8 inch) entire wheat tortillas or wraps

Headings

Join cilantro, vinegar, garlic, 1/2 teaspoon cumin and 1/4 teaspoon salt in a scaled down food processor; beat until finely hacked. With the engine running, gradually stream in oil. Move the vinaigrette to an enormous bowl. Add lettuce, radicchio and radishes and throw to cover.

Pound beans, stew powder, garlic powder, the leftover 1/2 teaspoon cumin and 1/4 teaspoon salt in a medium bowl.

Pound avocado with lime juice in a little bowl. Spread a portion of the pounded beans and avocado over every tortilla; top with the serving of mixed greens and roll up.

6. **Vegan Rice Bowls**

Prep Time:30 mins
Total Time:30 mins
Servings:4
Yield:4 servings

Ingredients

1. 1 medium yam, stripped whenever wanted, cut into 1-inch pieces
2. 3 tablespoons extra-virgin olive oil, separated
3. ½ teaspoon salt, separated
4. ½ teaspoon ground pepper, separated
5. 2 tablespoons tahini
6. 2 tablespoons water
7. 1 tablespoon lemon juice
8. 1 little clove garlic, minced
9. 2 cups cooked quinoa
10. 1 15-ounce can chickpeas, washed
11. 1 firm ready avocado, diced
12. ¼ cup cleaved new cilantro or parsley

Bearings

Preheat the stove to 425 degrees F.

Throw yam with 1 tablespoon oil and 1/4 teaspoon each salt and pepper in a medium bowl. Move to a rimmed baking sheet. Broil, blending once, until delicate, 15 to 18 minutes.

In the meantime, whisk the leftover 2 tablespoons oil, tahini, water, lemon juice, garlic and the excess 1/4 teaspoon each salt and pepper in a little bowl.

To serve, partition quinoa among 4 dishes. Top with equivalent measures of yam, chickpeas and avocado. Sprinkle with the tahini sauce. Sprinkle with parsley (or cilantro).

7. **Stuffed Sweet Potato With Hummus Recipe**

Prep Time:15 mins
Additional Time:5 mins
Total Time:20 mins
Servings:1
Yield:1 stuffed sweet potato

Ingredients

1. 1 enormous yam, scoured
2. ¾ cup slashed kale
3. 1 cup canned dark beans, flushed
4. ¼ cup hummus
5. 2 tablespoons water

Headings

Prick yam done with a fork. For seven to ten minutes, on High, heat until thoroughly done.

In the meantime, wash kale and channel, permitting water to stick to the leaves. Place in a medium pan; cover and cook over medium-high intensity, mixing on more than one occasion, until shriveled. Add beans; add a tablespoon or two of water in the event that the pot is dry. Keep cooking, uncovered, blending once in a while, until the combination is steaming hot, 1 to 2 minutes.

Part the yam open and top with the kale and bean combination. Consolidate hummus and 2 tablespoons of water in a little dish. Add extra water depending on the situation to arrive at the desired consistency. Shower the hummus dressing over the stuffed yam.

8. Quick Lentil Salmon Salad

Cook Time:30 mins
Total Time:30 mins
Servings:4
Yield:4 servings

Ingredients

1. ¾ cup earthy colored lentils
2. ½ cup slashed red onion in addition to 1/4 cup meagerly cut, partitioned
3. 2 cloves garlic, minced
4. ¾ teaspoon salt
5. ¼ cup extra-virgin olive oil
6. 3 tablespoons red-wine vinegar
7. ¾ teaspoon dried thyme
8. ¼ teaspoon ground pepper
9. 1 15-ounce can salmon, depleted
10. 1 cup carrot strips
11. 1 cup cut celery
12. 4 lemon wedges for serving

Headings

Bring a medium-sized pan of water to a boil. Add lentils and slashed onion, diminish intensity to keep an enthusiastic stew and cook until the lentils are simply delicate, 11 to 13 minutes. Channel well.

In the meantime, squash garlic and salt into a glue with the side of a culinary expert's blade (or a fork). Move to a medium bowl and speed in oil, vinegar, thyme and pepper.

Eliminate any skin or potentially bones from salmon; piece the salmon into a huge bowl. Add cut onion, carrot and 3 tablespoons of the dressing; delicately throw to cover. Add celery and the lentils to the excess dressing; tenderly mix to consolidate. Split the lentils between 4 dishes, top with the salmon plate of mixed greens and present with lemon wedges.

9. Cucumber Salad Hummus & Pita Bents

Active Time:15 mins
Total Time:15 mins
Servings:1
Yield:1 serving

Ingredients

1. ¼ cup chickpeas, washed
2. ¼ cup diced cucumber
3. ¼ cup diced tomato
4. 1 tablespoon diced olives
5. 1 tablespoon disintegrated feta cheddar
6. 1 tablespoon hacked new parsley
7. ½ teaspoon extra-virgin olive oil
8. 1 teaspoon red-wine vinegar
9. 3 ounces barbecued turkey bosom tenderloin or chicken bosom
10. 1 cup grapes
11. 1 entire wheat pita bread, quartered
12. 2 tablespoons hummus

Bearings

Throw chickpeas, cucumber, tomato, olives, feta, parsley, oil and vinegar together in a medium bowl. Pack in a medium-sized compartment.

Place turkey (or chicken) in a medium compartment.
Pack grapes and pita in little compartments and hummus in a plunge size holder.

Chapter 4: Delicious Dinner Recipes

1. Minestra Maritata

Active Time:20 mins
Total Time:20 mins
Servings:6
Yield:9 cups

Ingredients
1. 4 tablespoons extra-virgin olive oil, partitioned
2. 1 ⅓ cups cleaved yellow onion
3. ⅔ cup cleaved carrot
4. ⅔ cup cleaved celery
5. 2 tablespoons minced garlic
6. 6 cups unsalted chicken stock
7. 6 ounces orzo, ideally entire wheat
8. 1 ½ tablespoons cleaved new oregano
9. ½ teaspoon genuine salt
10. 24 cooked chicken meatballs (12 ounces), like Simple Chicken Meatballs (see related recipe)
11. 4 cups child spinach
12. ¼ cup ground Parmesan cheddar

Headings
Heat 1 tablespoon of oil in an enormous pot or Dutch stove over medium-high intensity. Add onion, carrot, celery and garlic; cook, blending incidentally, until the onion is clear, 4 to 5 minutes.

Add stock, cover and heat to the point of boiling. Add orzo, oregano and salt; cover and cook, blending incidentally, until the orzo is simply delicate, around 9 minutes.

Mix in meatballs and spinach; cook until the meatballs are warmed through and the spinach is withered, 2 to 4 minutes.

Serve sprinkled with cheddar and showered with the excess 3 tablespoons of oil.

2. **Spinach & Artichoke Dip Pasta**

Active Time:20 mins
Total Time:20 mins
Servings:4
Yield:4 servings

Ingredients
8 ounces entire wheat rotini
1 (5 ounce) bundle child spinach, generally slashed
4 ounces diminished fat cream cheddar, cut into pieces
¾ cup diminished fat milk
½ cup ground Parmesan cheddar, in addition to something else for decorate, whenever wanted
2 teaspoons garlic powder
¼ teaspoon ground pepper
1 (14 ounce) can artichoke hearts, flushed, crushed dry and cleaved (see Tip)

Headings
Bring a large saucepan of water to a rolling boil.

As directed by the bundle bearings, cook the pasta.

Join spinach and 1 tablespoon water in an enormous pan over medium intensity. Cook, blending once in a while, until recently withered, around 2 minutes. Move to a little bowl.

Add cream cheddar and milk to the container; speed until the cream cheddar is softened.

Add Parmesan, garlic powder and pepper; cook, racing until thickened and foaming.

Channel however much fluid as could reasonably be expected from the spinach. Mix the depleted spinach into the sauce, alongside artichokes and the pasta. Cook until warmed through.

Tip
On the off chance that you can find frozen artichoke hearts, they likewise function admirably in this recipe. Defrost prior to utilizing.

3. Hearty Chickpea & Spinach Stew

Prep Time:20 mins
Additional Time:10 mins
Total Time:30 mins
Servings:4
Yield:8 cups

Ingredients

2 (15 ounce) jars low-sodium chickpeas, flushed, partitioned
1 tablespoon olive oil
12 ounces 93%-lean ground turkey
½ teaspoon dried oregano
½ teaspoon fennel seeds, squashed
½ teaspoon squashed red pepper
1 medium onion, slashed (1 cup)
2 medium carrots, diced (3/4 cup)
Half a teaspoon of garlic powder or four chopped garlic cloves
3 tablespoons tomato glue
1 (32 ounce) container low-sodium chicken stock (4 cups)
¼ teaspoon ground pepper
⅛ teaspoon salt
3 cups IQF (independently fast frozen) spinach (8 oz.)
¼ cup ground Parmesan cheddar (Discretionary)

Headings

Pound 1 can chickpeas with a potato masher or fork. Put away.

Heat oil in an enormous pot over medium-high intensity.

Add turkey, oregano, fennel seeds and crushed red pepper.

Cook, disintegrating with a wooden spoon, until the turkey is at this point not pink, 2 to 3 minutes. Add the garlic (or garlic powder), onion, and carrots. Cook, mixing frequently, until relaxed and fragrant, 3 to 4 minutes. Add tomato glue. Cook, mixing, for 30 seconds.

Add stock, the crushed and entire chickpeas, pepper and salt to the pot. Cover and bring to a stew. Lessen intensity to medium and cook, covered, at a lively stew until the vegetables are delicate and the flavors have mixed, around 10 minutes.

Add spinach and increment intensity to medium-high, Cook, blending, until the spinach is warmed through, 1 to 2 minutes. Spoon the soup into bowls. Embellish each present with 1 tablespoon Parmesan, whenever wanted.

Tip
Separately fast frozen (IQF) spinach makes this recipe a breeze. In the event that you can't find it, utilize a frozen 10-ounce block of spinach. Cook as per the bundle headings, then add to the soup in step 4.

4. **20- Minute Balsamic Mushroom & Spinach Pasta**

Active Time:20 mins
Total Time:20 mins
Servings:6

Ingredients
1. 8 ounces entire wheat fettuccine or linguine
2. 4 tablespoons extra-virgin olive oil, separated
3. 1 pound cremini mushrooms, cut (around 6 cups)
4. 1 ½ tablespoons daintily cut garlic
5. 3 ounces child spinach (around 3 cups)
6. 3 tablespoons balsamic vinegar
7. 2 teaspoons Worcestershire sauce, ideally veggie lover
8. ¾ teaspoon salt
9. ½ teaspoon ground pepper
10. ¼ cup hacked new basil
11. 6 tablespoons hacked roasted unsalted pistachios

Bearings
Heat a huge pot of water to the point of boiling. Cook pasta as per bundle bearings. Channel, saving 1/4 cup cooking water.

In the meantime, heat 2 tablespoons of oil in a huge nonstick skillet over medium-high intensity. Add mushrooms; cook, mixing incidentally, until very much seared, around 10 minutes. Mix in garlic; cook, blending continually, until fragrant, around 30 seconds. Mix in spinach; cook, blending continually, until shriveled, around 1 moment.

Diminish intensity to medium-low; mix in balsamic vinegar, Worcestershire, salt, pepper and the excess 2 tablespoons oil. Add the pasta and throw to cover. Mix in the saved 1/4 cup cooking water. Eliminate from heat.

Mix in basil and sprinkle with pistachios.

5. **Kale & Avocado Salad With Blueberries & Edamame**

Prep Time:20 mins
Total Time:20 mins
Servings:4
Yield:8 cups

Ingredients

6 cups stemmed and coarsely hacked wavy kale
1 avocado, diced
1 cup blueberries
1 cup split yellow cherry tomatoes
1 cup cooked shelled edamame
¼ cup cut almonds, toasted (see Tip)
½ cup disintegrated goat cheddar (2 ounces)
¼ cup olive oil
3 tablespoons lemon juice
1 tablespoon minced chives
1 ½ teaspoons honey

Instructions

Place kale in a huge bowl and, utilizing your hands, back rub to mellow the leaves. Add avocado, blueberries, tomatoes, edamame, almonds, and goat cheddar.

Consolidate oil, lemon juice, chives, honey, mustard, and salt in a little bowl or in a container with a tight-fitting cover. Whisk or shake well.

Shower the vinaigrette over the plate of mixed greens and throw to join.

Tips

To make ahead: Wash, stem, and cleave kale, cook edamame, toast almonds, and make vinaigrette (Stage 2) as long as 1 day ahead and refrigerate.
Tip: To toast cut (or hacked) nuts, place in a little dry skillet and cook over medium-low intensity, mixing continually, until fragrant, 2 to 4 minutes.

6. **One Pot Lentil & Vegetable Soup With Permesan**

Active Time:15 mins
Total Time:40 mins
Servings:6

Ingredients

1. 2 tablespoons extra-virgin olive oil
2. 3 cups new or frozen hacked onion, carrot and celery blend
3. 4 cloves garlic, hacked
4. 4 cups low-sodium vegetable or chicken stock
5. 1 ½ cups green or earthy colored lentils
6. 1 (15-ounce) can unsalted diced tomatoes, undrained
7. 2 teaspoons finely hacked new thyme
8. ½ teaspoon salt
9. ½ teaspoon ground pepper
10. ½ teaspoon crushed red pepper
11. ½ cup ground Parmesan cheddar
12. Parmesan skin (discretionary)
13. 3 cups stuffed generally cleaved lacinato kale
14. 1 ½ tablespoons red-wine vinegar
15. Hacked new level leaf parsley for decorate

Bearings

Heat oil in a Dutch stove or enormous pot over medium intensity. Add onion, carrot and celery blend; cook, mixing incidentally, until relaxed, 6 to 10 minutes. Add garlic; cook, mixing frequently, until fragrant, around 30 seconds.

7. **Egg Drop Soup With Instant Noodles, Spinach & Scallions**

Prep time:15 mins

Total Time:15 mins

Servings:1
Yield:2 cups

Ingredients

1. 2 cups water
2. ½ (3 ounce) bundle rice-noodle soup blend, like Thai Kitchen Garlic and Vegetable
3. 1 huge egg
4. 1 cup child spinach
5. 1 scallion, cut

Instructions

Heat water to the point of boiling in a little pot. Mix in portions of the flavoring parcel (dispose of the rest to save for another utilization). Add noodles and cook until delicate, around 3 minutes. Diminish intensity to keep a stew.

Whisk egg in a little bowl. Gradually empty the egg into the stewing soup, mixing continually. Crease in spinach until recently withered, around 30 seconds. Move to a bowl and sprinkle with scallion.

8. **Salt & Vinegar Sheets Pan Chicken & Brussels Sprouts**

Prep Time:20 mins
Additional Time:25 mins
Total Time:45 mins
Servings:4
Yield:4 servings

Ingredients

1. 1 ½ pounds bone-in, skin-on chicken bosoms
2. 3 tablespoons extra-virgin olive oil, partitioned
3. 1 teaspoon genuine salt, isolated
4. ½ teaspoon ground pepper, partitioned
5. 1 ½ pounds Brussels grows, managed and split or quartered if enormous
6. Two medium red onions, sliced into wedges measuring 1/2 inch
7. 6 tablespoons malt vinegar or sherry vinegar
8. ½ teaspoon dried dill
9. ½ teaspoon garlic powder
10. ½ teaspoon onion powder
11. ¼ teaspoon sugar

Bearings

Preheat the stove to 450 degrees F.

Cut chicken bosoms into 4 equivalent segments. Brush with 1 tablespoon of oil and sprinkle with 1/4 teaspoon each salt and pepper. Throw Brussels fledglings and onions in a huge bowl with the leftover 2 tablespoons oil and 1/4 teaspoon each salt and pepper. Orchestrate the vegetables and the chicken in a solitary layer on a rimmed baking sheet.

Broil until a moment to read the thermometer embedded in the thickest piece of a bosom without contacting bone registers 160 degrees F and the vegetables are delicate, 20 to 25 minutes.

In the meantime, blend vinegar, dill, garlic powder, onion powder, sugar and the excess 1/2 teaspoon salt in a little microwave-safe bowl. Microwave on High until the salt and sugar break up, around 30 seconds.

Shower the vinegar blend over the chicken and vegetables and dish for 5 minutes more. Move the chicken to a serving platter and mix the vegetables on the dish. Serve the vegetables with the chicken.

9. **Buffalo Cauliflower Tacos**

Active Time:20 mins
Total Time:40 mins
Servings:6

Ingredients
1. 6 cups cauliflower florets
2. ½ cup Bison style hot sauce
3. 2 tablespoons extra-virgin olive oil, in addition to 1 1/2 teaspoons, separated
4. ⅓ cup destroyed cheddar
5. 1 ½ cups new corn pieces
6. 1 ½ cups finely destroyed romaine lettuce
7. 1 medium avocado, cut
8. 12 (6-inch) corn tortillas, warmed
9. ½ cup farm dressing

Bearings
Place rack in upper third of stove; preheat to 425°F. Line a huge rimmed baking sheet with material paper.

Consolidate cauliflower, Hot sauce and 2 tablespoons oil in an enormous bowl; throw well to cover. Spread in an even layer on the pre-arranged baking sheet. Cook until the cauliflower begins to brown and is practically delicate, 12 to 14 minutes. Eliminate from broiler and sprinkle equitably with cheddar. Keep simmering until the cauliflower is delicate, 8 to 10 minutes. Put away until prepared to serve.

Heat an enormous nonstick skillet over medium-high intensity. Add corn and the excess 1 1/2 teaspoons oil; cook, blending periodically, until the corn is rankled and roasted, around 5 minutes. Eliminate from heat.

Partition the cauliflower, lettuce, corn and avocado equally among warm tortillas. Shower equitably with farm dressing. Serve right away.

Tips
Equipment: Parchment paper

10. **Roasted Root Veggies & Green Over Spiced Lentils**

Prep Time:20 mins
Additional Time:25 mins
Total Time:45 mins
Servings:2
Yield:2 servings

Ingredients
Lentils
1 ½ cups water
½ cup dark beluga lentils or French green lentils (see Tip)
1 teaspoon garlic powder
½ teaspoon ground coriander
½ teaspoon ground cumin
¼ teaspoon ground allspice
¼ teaspoon genuine salt
⅛ teaspoon sumac (discretionary)
2 tablespoons lemon juice
1 teaspoon extra-virgin olive oil
Vegetables
1 tablespoon extra-virgin olive oil
1 clove garlic, crushed
1 1/2 cups cooked root vegetables (see related recipes)
2 cups hacked kale or beet greens
1 teaspoon ground coriander
⅛ teaspoon ground pepper
Touch of fit salt
2 tablespoons tahini or low-fat plain yogurt
New parsley for embellish

Bearings
To get ready lentils: Join water, lentils, garlic powder, 1/2 teaspoon coriander, cumin, allspice, 1/4 teaspoon salt and sumac (if utilizing) in a medium pot. Heat to the point of

boiling. Decrease intensity to keep a stew, cover and cook until delicate, 25 to 30 minutes.

Uncover and keep stewing until the fluid decreases somewhat, around 5 minutes more. Channel. Mix in lemon juice and 1 teaspoon oil.

In the meantime, to get ready vegetables: Intensity oil in
a huge skillet over medium intensity. Cook the garlic for one to two minutes, or until fragrant. Add roasted root vegetables and cook, blending frequently, until warmed through, 2 to 4 minutes. Mix in kale (or beet greens) and cook until recently shriveled, 2 to 3 minutes. Mix in coriander, pepper and salt.

Serve the vegetables over the lentils, finished off with tahini (or yogurt). Embellish with parsley, whenever wanted.

Tip
We like dark beluga lentils or French green lentils rather than earthy colored when we need lentils that hold their shape (rather than separating) when cooked. Search for them in regular food varieties stores and a few general stores.

Chapter 5: Satisfying Snacks

1. Cinnamon- sugar Roasted Chickpeas

Prep Time:5 mins
Additional Time:50 mins
Total Time:55 mins
Servings:4
Yield:1 cup

Ingredients
1 (15 ounce) can chickpeas, flushed
1 tablespoon sugar
1 teaspoon ground cinnamon
⅛ teaspoon ground pepper
1 tablespoon avocado oil

Headings
Position rack in the upper third of broiler; preheat to 450 degrees F.

Smear chickpeas dry. Spread on a rimmed baking sheet.

Prepare for 10 minutes. In the meantime blend sugar, cinnamon and pepper in a little bowl.

Move the chickpeas to a medium bowl and throw with oil and the cinnamon-sugar combination. Get back to the baking sheet and heat, blending once, until carmelized and crunchy, 15 to 20 minutes more. Let cool on the baking sheet for 15 minutes.

Tips
To make ahead: Store in a water/air proof compartment for as long as a day.

2. Almond-stuffed Dates

Cook Time:5 mins
Total Time:5 mins
Servings:1
Yield:1 serving

Ingredients
2 pitted Medjool dates
2 salted entire almonds
¼ teaspoon orange zing

Headings
Stuff each date with an almond and roll in orange zing.

3. Sriracha- Buffalo Cauliflower Bites

Active Time:10 mins
Additional Time:20 mins
Total Time:25 mins
Servings:6
Yield:6 servings

Ingredients

1. 8 cups 1 1/2-inch cauliflower florets
2. 2 tablespoons extra-virgin olive oil
3. ¼ teaspoon genuine salt
4. 2 tablespoons hot sauce, like Straightforward's RedHot
5. 1-2 tablespoons Sriracha
6. 1 tablespoon spread, liquefied
7. 1 tablespoon lemon juice

Bearings

Preheat the stove to 450°F. Cover a huge rimmed baking sheet with a cooking shower.

Throw cauliflower, oil and salt in a huge bowl. Spread on the pre-arranged baking sheet; save the bowl. Cook the cauliflower until it's beginning to mellow and brown on the base, around 15 minutes.

In the meantime, consolidate hot sauce, Sriracha to taste, margarine and lemon juice in the enormous bowl. Add the simmered cauliflower and throw to cover. Return the cauliflower to the baking sheet and keep simmering until hot, around 5 minutes more.

4. **Cranberry - Almond Granola Bars**

Prep Time:20 mins
Additional Time:1 hr 10 mins
Total Time:1 hr 30 mins
Servings:1
Yield:24 bars

Ingredients
3 cups dated moved oats
1 cup fresh earthy colored rice cereal
1 cup dried cranberries
½ cup almonds, toasted and slashed
½ cup walnuts, toasted and cleaved
¼ teaspoon salt
⅔ cup earthy colored rice syrup or light corn syrup
½ cup smooth almond margarine
1 teaspoon vanilla concentrate

Headings
Preheat broiler to 325 degrees F. Line a 9-by-13-inch baking container with material paper, leaving additional material looming north of different sides. Gently cover the material with a cooking splash.

Join oats, rice grain, cranberries, almonds, walnuts and salt in an enormous bowl.

Join rice syrup (or corn syrup), almond spread and vanilla in a microwave-safe bowl. Microwave for 30 seconds (or intensity in a pan over medium intensity for 1 moment).

Add to the dry fixings and mix until uniformly consolidated. Move to the pre-arranged container and immovably press into the skillet with the rear of a spatula.

For chewier bars, heat until scarcely beginning to variety around the edge yet delicate in the center, 20 to 25 minutes. For crunchier bars, heat until brilliant brown around the edge and fairly firm in the center, 30 to 35 minutes. (Both will in any case be delicate when warm and solidify as they cool.)

Give cool access to the search for gold minutes, then, at that point, utilizing the material to help you, lift out of the dish onto a cutting board (it will in any case be delicate). Cut into 24 bars, then, at that point, let cool totally without isolating the bars, around 30 minutes more. When cool, separate into bars.

Tips
To make ahead: Independently wrap hermetically sealed and store at room temperature for as long as multi week.
Gear: Material paper

5. **Everything Seasoned Almonds**

Active Time:5 mins
Total Time:1 hr 20 mins
Servings:12

Ingredients
1 huge egg white
3 tablespoons all that bagel preparing, ground
3 cups crude unsalted almonds

Headings
Preheat broiler to 250°F.

Whisk egg white and prepare in a medium bowl. Add almonds and throw to cover. Spread in an even layer on an enormous rimmed baking sheet.

Heat, mixing like clockwork, until dry, around 45 minutes. Let cool totally prior to putting away, around 30 minutes.

Tips
To make ahead: Store in a sealed shut holder for as long as about fourteen days.

6. Fig & Honey Yogurt

Cook Time:5 mins
Total Time:5 mins
Servings:1
Yield:1 serving

Ingredients

1. ⅔ cup low-fat plain yogurt
2. 3 dried figs, cut
3. 2 teaspoons honey

Bearings

Place yogurt in a bowl and top with figs and honey.

Chapter 6: Guilt- Free Dessert

1. Lemon- Blueberry Poke Cake

Active Time:25 mins
Total Time:1 hr 40 mins
Servings:10

Ingredients

1. 1 ¼ cups sugar, isolated
2. ½ cup impartial oil, like avocado or light olive oil
3. ⅓ cup low-fat plain yogurt
4. 2 tablespoons lemon zing
5. 1 teaspoon vanilla concentrate
6. 2 enormous eggs
7. 1 cup entire wheat baked good flour or white entire wheat flour
8. ¾ cup regular baking flour
9. 1 teaspoon baking powder
10. ½ teaspoon baking pop
11. ¼ teaspoon salt
12. 1 ½ cups new blueberries
13. 5 tablespoons lemon juice

Headings

Preheat broiler to 350°F. Cover a 9-by-5-inch portion skillet with cooking splash.

Beat 3/4 cup sugar, oil, yogurt, lemon zing and vanilla in an enormous bowl with an electric blender on medium speed until consolidated. Add eggs and beat until totally joined.

Whisk cake flour (or white entire wheat flour), regular flour, baking powder, baking pop and salt in a medium bowl. Add the flour combination and blueberries to the wet blend and overlap with a wooden spoon until recently joined. Move to the pre-arranged skillet.

58

Heat until brilliant and a wooden pick embedded in the middle tells the truth, around 60 minutes. Give cool for 5 minutes, access the container, then run a blade around the edges to release the cake. Transform onto a cooling rack, then, at that point, return to the portion container.

Whisk lemon juice with the leftover 1/2 cup sugar in a little bowl until smooth. Utilizing a metal or wooden stick, jab 1 1/2-inch-profound openings all around the cake.

Spoon the frosting all around the outer layer of the cake, allowing it to leak down the edges and into the openings.

Let represent 15 minutes then, utilizing a pie server or adaptable spatula, eliminate the cake to the cooling rack.

Cool totally prior to cutting.

2. **Strawberry - Chocolate Greek Yogurt Bark**

Active Time:10 mins
Additional Time:3 hrs
Total Time:3 hrs 10 mins
Servings:32
Yield:32 pieces

Ingredients

1. 3 cups entire milk plain Greek yogurt
2. ¼ cup unadulterated maple syrup or honey
3. 1 teaspoon vanilla concentrate
4. 1 ½ cups cut strawberries
5. ¼ cup small scale chocolate chips

Headings

Line an enormous rimmed baking sheet with material paper.

In a medium bowl, combine yogurt, vanilla, and maple syrup (or honey).. Spread on the pre-arranged baking sheet into a 10-by-15-inch square shape. Disperse the strawberries on top and sprinkle with chocolate chips.

Freeze until extremely firm, no less than 3 hours. To serve, Cut or split into 32 pieces to serve.

3. Lemon- Blueberry Nice Cream

Active Time:10 mins
Total Time:10 mins
Servings:4

Ingredients

3 medium ready bananas, cut and frozen
¼ cup lemon juice
¼ teaspoon vanilla concentrate
¼ cup cold water, depending on the situation
¾ cup frozen blueberries

Headings

Place frozen banana cuts, lemon juice and vanilla in a food processor. Process until smooth, adding cold water to relax the blend, if fundamental. Move to a bowl; mix in frozen blueberries. Serve right away or store in a hermetically sealed holder in the cooler for as long as several months.

To make ahead
Store in a water/air proof compartment in the cooler for as long as multi month.

4. **Apple Coffee Cake**

Prep Time:20 mins
Additional Time:1 hr
Total Time:1 hr 20 mins
Servings:16
Yield:16 squares

Ingredients
Baking splash with flour
1 ¼ cups light earthy colored sugar, partitioned
¾ cup unsalted spread, mellowed, separated
¼ cup granulated sugar
3 huge eggs
3 teaspoons vanilla concentrate, partitioned
2 ¼ cups white entire wheat flour, partitioned
3 teaspoons ground cinnamon, partitioned
1 teaspoon baking pop
1 teaspoon baking powder
½ teaspoon salt
1 cup plain entire milk Greek yogurt
2 medium Granny Smith apples, stripped and cut into 1/2-inch solid shapes (around 3 cups)
½ cup dated moved oats
¼ cup hacked walnuts
½ cup confectioners' sugar
1 tablespoon entire milk

Bearings
Preheat stove to 350 degrees F. Coat a 9-inch-square baking dish (no less than 2 1/4 inches down) with baking splash.

Consolidate 3/4 cup earthy colored sugar, 1/2 cup spread and granulated sugar in the bowl of a stand blender fitted with an oar connection. Beat on medium speed until light and soft, around 3 minutes. Add eggs, 1 all at once, beating on low speed just until mixed after every option.

Add 2 teaspoons vanilla; beat on low until mixed.

Whisk 1 3/4 cups flour and 2 teaspoons cinnamon in a medium bowl. Add baking pop, baking powder and salt; rush to consolidate. Add the flour combination to the spread blend on the other hand with yogurt, starting and finishing with the flour combination and beating on low speed just until mixed after every option. Overlap in apples.

Join oats, walnuts and the excess 1/2 cup flour, 1/2 cup earthy colored sugar and 1 teaspoon cinnamon in a medium bowl. Add the leftover 1/4 cup spread and utilize your fingers to work it into the combination until mixed and brittle.

Spread a portion of the hitter in an even layer in the pre-arranged baking dish. Sprinkle equally with around 50% of the oat-walnut combination. Spoon the leftover player on top and spread it to the edges of the skillet. Top with the leftover oat-walnut blend.

Prepare until a wooden pick embedded in the focal point of the cake tells the truth, 45 to 55 minutes. If vital, freely cover with foil after around 30 minutes to forestall extreme carmelizing. Give cool access the dish on a wire rack for 15 minutes.

Whisk confectioners' sugar, milk and the leftover 1 teaspoon vanilla in a little bowl until smooth. Shower over the warm cake. Serve warm, or cool totally, around 45 minutes. Cut into 16 squares.

Tips
To make ahead: Cover and store at room temperature for as long as 1 day.

5. **Naturally Red Velvet Doughnuts**

Prep Time:45 mins
Additional Time:15 mins
Total Time:1 hr
Servings:12
Yield:12 doughnuts

Ingredients
Doughnuts
¾ cup slashed cooked stripped beets

¾ cup granulated sugar

1 enormous egg yolk, at room temperature

½ teaspoon fit salt

¾ cup buttermilk

1 tablespoon vanilla concentrate

1 cup regular baking flour

1 cup white entire wheat flour

¼ cup freeze-dried pomegranate powder (see Tip)

2 ½ tablespoons unsweetened normal cocoa powder (not Dutch-process), filtered

1 ½ teaspoons baking powder

⅓ cup safflower or canola oil

3 tablespoons unsalted margarine, mellowed

Icing
1 cup confectioners' sugar

1 tablespoon decreased fat cream cheddar, mellowed

2 teaspoons lemon juice

¼ teaspoon vanilla concentrate

Bearings
To get ready doughnuts: Preheat stove to 350 degrees F. Liberally cover 12 standard-size donut dish cups with cooking splash.

Process beets in a food processor until finely hacked, scratching down the sides as required. Add granulated sugar, egg yolk and salt; process until totally smooth, 3 to 4 minutes. Add buttermilk and 1 tablespoon vanilla; process, scratching down the sides depending on the situation, until equally integrated.

Consolidate regular flour, entire wheat flour, pomegranate powder, cocoa and baking powder in a medium bowl.

Beat oil and spread in a huge bowl with an electric blender until completely mixed. With the blender on low speed, on the other hand blend the dry fixings and the wet fixings into the oil combination, beginning and finishing with the dry fixings and scratching down the sides on a case by case basis, until recently consolidated. Split the hitter between the pre-arranged donut cups.

Heat until a toothpick embedded in the thickest piece of a donut in the focal point of the container confesses all, 13 to 16 minutes. Allow the skillet to cool for ten minutes on a wire rack.
. Eliminate the doughnuts from the skillet, modifying so the bottoms become the tops, and let cool totally on the rack.

To plan icing: Beat confectioners' sugar, cream cheddar, lemon juice and vanilla in a medium bowl with an electric blender until smooth. Plunge the doughnuts in the frosting. Let represent around 5 minutes so the icing can set.

Tips
To make ahead: Refrigerate water/air proof for as long as 2 days or freeze for as long as multi month. Warm through until room temperature before serving.
Hardware: Two 6-cup donut container
Tip: Freeze-Dried Organic product for Food Shading
Freeze-dried natural products have all their water eliminated in an intensity free, vacuum process that likewise safeguards tones, keeps enhances new and fruity and makes a brittle surface (in contrast to the rough, generally dried ones). Ground into powder, they're great for shading.
Where to Purchase: Both freeze-dried leafy foods ground powders are promptly accessible. Search for them at the grocery store with other dried natural product or online at amazon.com.
To Set them up: Drudgery freeze-dried organic products in a food processor until they become a fine powder. (Assuming you find dried organic products previously powdered, there's a compelling reason you need to crush them.)

6. **Oatmeal Cookies Fruit Pizza**

Prep Time:30 mins
Additional Time:2 hrs 15 mins
Total Time:2 hrs 45 mins
Servings:10
Yield:10 servings

Ingredients
Crust
1 ½ cups outdated moved oats
1 cup white entire wheat flour
½ teaspoon ground cinnamon
½ teaspoon baking pop
¼ teaspoon baking powder
¼ teaspoon salt
1 enormous egg
⅔ cup pressed light earthy colored sugar
⅓ cup canola oil
½ teaspoon vanilla concentrate
Beating
8 ounces diminished fat cream cheddar, at room temperature
½ cup low-fat plain Greek yogurt
3 tablespoons filtered confectioners' sugar
1 teaspoon vanilla concentrate
¾ cup cut strawberries
1 kiwi, stripped, divided and cut
¼ cup blueberries

Headings
Preheat broiler to 375 degrees F. Line an enormous baking sheet with material paper.

To plan hull: Join oats, flour, cinnamon, baking pop, baking powder and salt in a medium bowl. Join egg, earthy colored sugar, oil and 1/2 teaspoon vanilla in another medium bowl. Add the wet fixings to the dry fixings and mix to join. (The combination will be dry.) Turn the mixture out onto the pre-arranged baking sheet and press into a 10-inch circle.

Prepare the outside layer until it is brilliant around the edges, around 20 minutes. Allow to cool to room temperature on the baking sheet.

To plan vesting: Beat cream cheddar, yogurt, confectioners' sugar and vanilla in a medium bowl with an electric blender until smooth. Spread the combination equally over the cooled outside. Gorgeously top with strawberries, kiwi and blueberries.

Tips
To make ahead: Plan to treat the hull (Stages 1-3) and store water/air proof for as long as 2 days.
Hardware: Material paper

Chapter 7: Refreshing Beverages

1. Easy Turmeric Tea

PREP: 5 minutes

COOK: 15 minutes

TOTAL: 20minutes

SERVINGS: 2 servings

Ingredients

- 2 cups water
  - 2 tablespoons lemon juice
  - ½ teaspoon ground turmeric
  - squeeze newly ground dark pepper
  - 2 teaspoons honey

Instructions

In a little pot, add water, turmeric, lemon squeeze, and dark pepper. Whisk together and heat over high intensity. At the point when the tea simply begins to bubble, turn the intensity down to low and stew for 10 minutes.

When the tea is done stewing, switch off the intensity, add the honey, and let the tea cool briefly.

Empty the tea into a mug through a sifter to eliminate the dark pepper and appreciate.

2. Green Smoothie

PREP: 5minutes

TOTAL: 5minutes

SERVINGS: 2 servings

Ingredients

- 1 ½ cup milk (dairy or sans dairy)
- ☐
- 2 cups child spinach
- ☐
- 1 frozen banana
- ☐
- 1 apple
- ☐
- ¼ avocado

Guidelines

Add each of the fixings to a blender and mix on high for 30 seconds, or until velvety.

Tips

Make sure to hold up your bananas somewhat early! I cut my bananas down the middle and afterward store them in a Stasher pack in the cooler.

3. Anti- Inflammatory Golden Tonic

Prep Time:10 mins
Additional Time:1 hr 15 mins
Total Time:1 hr 25 mins
Servings:4
Yield:4 cups

Ingredients

1. 2 cups separated water
2. 2 sacks green tea
3. 5 twigs new thyme, gently swollen with the side of a blade
4. 1 (2 inch) piece stripped ginger, finely ground
5. 1 (2 inch) piece stripped turmeric, finely ground
6. 1 tablespoon honey, ideally manuka
7. 1 tablespoon crude unfiltered juice vinegar
8. Ice blocks
9. 2 cups chilled shimmering water
10. Lime wedges for serving

Headings

Carry sifted water to a delicate stew in a little pot over medium-high intensity. Add tea packs, thyme, ginger, turmeric, honey and vinegar, mixing to disintegrate the honey. Lessen intensity to low and allow the blend to soak for 15 minutes. Strain through a fine-network sifter into a bricklayer container. Refrigerate for 60 minutes.

Fill 4 glasses half loaded with ice. Partition the tonic blend equally among the glasses (around 1/2 cup tonic for every glass). Top each with 1/2 cup shimmering water. Present with a lime wedge, whenever wanted.

4. Sparkling Strawberry - Ginger Tonic

Active Time: 10 mins
Total Time: 10 mins
Servings: 6

Ingredients

1. 1 cup hulled strawberries (around 6 ounces), in addition to cut or potentially entire berries for decorate
2. 1 (1-liter) bottle shimmering pink lemonade
3. 2 (12 ounce) bottles ginger lager
4. Mint branches for decorate

Headings

Place strawberries in an enormous glass estimating cup; pound with a muddler or wooden spoon until extremely delicious. Move the combination to a fine-network sifter set over a bowl; press solidly to communicate however much squeeze as could reasonably be expected. (Save the solids for another utilization.)

Join the strawberry juice, lemonade and ginger lager in an enormous pitcher. Serve over ice in tall glasses. Decorate with cut as well as entire berries and mint twigs, whenever wanted.

5. **Elderberry Elixir Mocktail**

Active Time:5 mins
Total Time:5 mins
Servings:1

Ingredients

2 ounces newly pressed squeezed orange
1 ounce elderberry syrup (see Tip)
½ ounce newly crushed lemon juice
¼ teaspoon ground turmeric, or more to taste
Ice
Shimmering water
Orange cut for embellish

Bearings

Consolidate squeezed orange, elderberry syrup, lemon juice and turmeric in a mixed drink shaker.
Fill the shaker 3/4 full with ice.
Cover and shake until chilled, then, at that point, strain into a stone glass loaded up with ice. (On the other hand, for a layered look, shake the citrus juices and turmeric and strain into a glass loaded up with squashed ice. Shower the elderberry syrup over the ice.)

Top with shining water and enhancement with an orange cut, whenever wanted.

Tips

Tip: You can purchase elderberry syrup in supermarkets and on the web. One brand, Sambucol, is generally accessible in store supplement areas.

Week 1 Meal plan

Day1

- **Breakfast: Blueberry - Banana Overnight Oats**

Prep Time:10 mins
Additional Time:5 hrs 50 mins
Total Time:6 hrs
Servings:1
Yield:1 cups
Ingredients
½ cup unsweetened coconut milk beverage
½ cup antiquated oats (see Tip)
½ tablespoon chia seeds (Discretionary)
½ banana, crushed
1 teaspoon maple syrup
Touch of salt
½ cup new blueberries
1 tablespoon unsweetened chipped coconut

Bearings
Consolidate coconut milk, oats, chia seeds (if utilizing), banana, maple syrup and salt in a slight container and mix. Top with blueberries and coconut, whenever wanted. Cover and refrigerate for the time being.

Tips
Tip: Individuals with celiac infection or gluten responsiveness ought to utilize oats that are named "without gluten," as oats are in many cases cross-debased with wheat and grain.
To make ahead: Refrigerate for as long as 1 day.

- **Morning snack:** ½ cup of blackberries

- **Lunch**: Green salad with edamame & beets

Active Time:15 mins
Total Time:15 mins
Servings:1
Yield:1 serving

Ingredients

2 cups mixed salad greens
1 cup shelled edamame, defrosted
½ medium crude beet, stripped and destroyed (around 1/2 cup)
2 tablespoons red-wine vinegar
1 tablespoon cleaved new cilantro
1 tablespoon extra-virgin olive oil
⅛ teaspoon salt
Newly ground pepper to taste

Headings

Organize greens, edamame and beet on an enormous plate. Whisk vinegar, cilantro, oil, salt and pepper in a little bowl. Sprinkle one tablespoon of the dressing over the greens and throw delicately to cover. Sprinkle the excess dressing over the whole serving of mixed greens.

To make ahead
Refrigerate salad and dressing independently for as long as 2 days; whisk dressing prior to sprinkling over the serving of mixed greens.

- **Evening snack** : 2 tbsp Turmeric- Tahini Dip

Prep Time:10 mins
Total Time:10 mins
Servings:8
Ingredients

1. ½ cup tahini
2. ¼ cup rice vinegar
3. ¼ cup water
4. 1 tablespoon ground new ginger

5. 2 teaspoons ground turmeric
6. 1 teaspoon ground garlic
7. ½ teaspoon salt

Bearings

Whisk tahini, vinegar, water, ginger, turmeric, garlic and salt in a medium bowl until very much consolidated.

- **Dinner:** Roasted squash & apple with dried cherries & pepitas

Prep Time:15 mins
Additional Time:30 mins
Total Time:45 mins
Servings:5
Yield:5 servings

Ingredients

1 medium oak seed squash (around 1 1/2 pounds)
2 medium apples
3 tablespoons extra-virgin olive oil
¾ teaspoon ground cinnamon
½ teaspoon ground allspice
½ teaspoon ground coriander
½ teaspoon salt
½ teaspoon ground pepper
¼ cup dried cherries
¼ cup toasted pepitas

Instructions

Preheat broiler to 425 degrees F. Cover a rimmed baking sheet with a cooking shower.

Divide squash and scoop out the seeds. Center apples. Squash and apples should be cut into 1-inch wedges.Whisk oil, cinnamon, allspice, coriander, salt and pepper in an enormous bowl. Add the squash and apples and throw to cover. Spread on the pre-arranged container.

Cook until delicate, 25 to 30 minutes. Serve finished off with dried cherries and pepitas

Day 2

- **Breakfast:** Raspberry Kefir Power Smoothie

Prep Time:5 mins
Total Time:5 mins
Servings:1

Ingredients
1. ½ frozen banana
2. ½ cup raspberries, new or frozen
3. ⅓ cup low-fat plain kefir
4. 2 teaspoons regular peanut butter
5. ½ teaspoon flaxmeal
6. 1 tablespoon 1-2 tablespoons water

Instructions

Join banana, raspberries, kefir, peanut butter and flax meal in a blender. Process until smooth, adding water a tablespoon at once.

- **Morning snack:** ⅓ cup of blueberries

- **Lunch:** Vegan Superfood grain bowl

Active Time:15 mins
Total Time:15 mins
Servings:4
Yield:4 containers

Ingredients

1 (8 ounce) pocket microwavable quinoa
½ cup hummus
2 tablespoons lemon juice
1 (5 ounce) bundle child kale
1 (8 ounce) bundle refrigerated cooked entire child beets, cut (or 2 cups from self-service counter)

1 cup frozen shelled edamame, defrosted
1 medium avocado, cut
¼ cup unsalted toasted sunflower seeds

Instructions
Get ready quinoa as per bundle headings; put away to cool.
Join hummus and lemon juice in a little bowl. Meager with water to wanted dressing consistency. Split the dressing between 4 little fixing holders with covers and refrigerate.
Split child kale between 4 single-serving compartments with tops. Top each with 1/2 cup of the quinoa, 1/2 cup beets, 1/4 cup edamame and 1 tablespoon sunflower seeds.
At the point when prepared to eat, top with 1/4 avocado and the hummus dressing.

- **Evening snack**: ½ sliced cucumber seasoned with salt and pepper

- **Indian-style spiced cauliflower and chickpea salad for dinner.**
Prep Time:20 mins
Additional Time:20 mins
Total Time:40 mins
Servings:2
Yield:2 servings
Ingredients
1 tablespoon curry powder
1 tablespoon olive oil
¼ teaspoon salt
1 ½ cups cauliflower florets
1 cup canned no-salt-added garbanzo beans (chickpeas), washed and depleted
¾ cup 1/2-inch carrot cuts
¼ cup plain without fat yogurt
1 tablespoon lime juice
½ teaspoon dark pepper
½ teaspoon ground new ginger or 1/4 teaspoon ground ginger
½ teaspoon minced new jalapeño chile pepper (see Tip) (Discretionary)
1 tablespoon without fat milk (Discretionary)
2 cups torn red-tipped leaf lettuce
1 cup stuffed new Italian parsley
¼ cup daintily cut red onion
Instructions

Preheat broiler to 450 degrees F. In a medium bowl, join curry powder, olive oil and salt. Add the cauliflower, garbanzo bean and carrots; throw to cover. Spread combination in a 15x10x1-inch baking skillet. Cook 20 to 25 minutes or until vegetables are delicate, mixing once.

In the mean time, for dressing, in a little bowl, mix together the yogurt, lime squeeze and ginger and, whenever wanted, jalapeño pepper. If necessary, flimsy with milk to wanted consistency.

In an enormous bowl, consolidate broiled vegetables, lettuce, parsley and onion. Top with dressing; throw to cover.

Tips

Tip: Chile peppers contain oils that can aggravate your skin and eyes. Wear plastic or elastic gloves while working with them.

Day 3

- **Breakfast** :

1 cup low-fat plain Greek yogurt
1 1/2 Tbsp. slashed pecans
1/4 cup blueberries
1 cup green tea
Top yogurt with pecans and blueberries.

- **Morning snack:** ⅔ cup of raspberries

- **Lunch**: Sweet potato and cauliflower rice bowl

- **Dinner** : superfood chopped salad with salmon & creamy garlic dressing

Prep Time:30 mins
Total Time:30 mins
Servings:4
Yield:4 servings

Ingredients

1 pound salmon filet
½ cup low-fat plain yogurt
¼ cup mayonnaise
2 tablespoons lemon juice
2 tablespoons ground Parmesan cheddar
1 tablespoon finely slashed new parsley
1 tablespoon clipped new chives
2 teaspoons diminished sodium tamari or soy sauce
1 medium clove garlic, minced
¼ teaspoon ground pepper
8 cups slashed wavy kale
2 cups slashed broccoli
2 cups slashed red cabbage
2 cups finely diced carrots
½ cup sunflower seeds, toasted

Instructions

Organize a rack in the upper third of the stove. Preheat the grill too high. Line a baking sheet with foil.

Put salmon on the pre-arranged baking sheet, skin-side down. Sear, pivoting the dish from front to back once, until the salmon is murky in the middle, 8 to 12 minutes. Cut into 4 parts.

In the meantime, whisk yogurt, mayonnaise, lemon juice, Parmesan, parsley, chives, tamari (or soy sauce), garlic and pepper in a little bowl.

Join kale, broccoli, cabbage, carrots and sunflower seeds in an enormous bowl. Add 3/4 cup of the dressing and throw to cover. Split the serving of mixed greens between 4 supper plates and top each with a piece of salmon and around 1 tablespoon of the excess dressing.

Day 4

Breakfast: Cocoa - chia pudding with raspberry
Prep Time:10 mins
Additional Time:8 hrs
Total Time:8 hrs 10 mins
Servings:1
Yield:1 cup
Ingredients

½ cup almond milk, or any other nondairy milk, without sugar

2 tablespoons chia seeds
2 teaspoons unadulterated maple syrup
½ teaspoon unsweetened cocoa powder
¼ teaspoon vanilla concentrate
½ cup new raspberries, partitioned
1 tablespoon toasted cut almonds, partitioned
Instructions
Mix almond milk (or other nondairy milk), chia seeds, maple syrup, cocoa powder and vanilla together in a little bowl. Cover and refrigerate for no less than 8 hours and as long as 3 days.
At the point when prepared to serve, mix well. Spoon about a portion of the pudding into a serving glass (or bowl) and top with a portion of the raspberries and almonds. Add the remainder of the pudding and top with the leftover raspberries and almonds.
To make ahead
Refrigerate pudding (Stage 1) for as long as 3 days. Wrap up with Stage 2 not long prior to serving.

Morning snack: ½ cup of low fat Greek yogurt

Lunch: Mashed Chickpeas salad with dill & capers

Evening snack : 1 medium carrots cut into sticks

Dinner: Stuffed sweet potato with hummus recipe

Day 5

- **Breakfast:** Southwestern Waffles
- **Morning snack**: 1 cup of green tea
- **Lunch**: Quick lentil salmon salad
- **Evening snack**: ¾ cup sliced cucumber
- **Dinner**: Korean steak kimchi & cauliflower rice bowl

Prep Time:30 mins

Total Time:30 mins

Servings:4

Yield:8 cups

Ingredients

2 enormous eggs

4 tablespoons toasted sesame oil, isolated

6 cups riced cauliflower

2 scallions, cut, greens and whites isolated

1 tablespoon minced ginger

¼ teaspoon salt

1 pound sirloin steak, meagerly cut

¼ cup gochujang

2 tablespoons toasted sesame seeds

1 cup destroyed carrots

½ cup kimchi

1 ounce Cut radishes for decorate

Instructions

Bring a medium-sized pan of water to a boil using high heat. Set a bowl of ice water close to the oven. Utilizing a spoon, delicately lower eggs into the bubbling water. Lessen intensity to keep a quick stew. Cook for 7 minutes. Move the eggs to the ice shower and let cool for 5 minutes. Strip the eggs and cut down the middle.

In the meantime, heat 2 tablespoons of oil in a huge skillet over medium-high intensity. Add cauliflower, scallion whites, ginger and salt. Cook, mixing habitually, until the cauliflower is mellowed, around 5 minutes. Move to a bowl and cover to keep warm. Wash and dry the container.

Heat the excess 2 tablespoons of oil in the container over medium-high intensity. Add steak and cook, blending, until as of now not pink, 2 to 4 minutes. Eliminate from intensity and mix in gochujang and sesame seeds.

To collect, split the cauliflower between 4 dishes. Top with the steak, carrots, kimchi, around 50% of an egg, scallion greens and radishes, whenever wanted

Day 6

- **Breakfast**: Egg salad avocado toast
- **Morning snack**: 12 walnuts half
- **Lunch**: Cucumber, salad hummus & pita bents
- **Evening snack**: ½ ounces of dark chocolate
- **Dinner**: Blistered broccoli with garlic & chives

Prep Time:30 mins

Total Time:30 mins

Servings:4

Yield:4 servings

Ingredients

4 cups broccoli florets (see Tip)

2 tablespoons olive oil

2 cloves garlic, meagerly cut

¼ teaspoon squashed red pepper

1 teaspoon finely destroyed lemon strip

2 teaspoons lemon juice

⅛ teaspoon fine ocean salt

Headings

Heat an iron container or weighty skillet over medium-high intensity. Add broccoli; cook around 10 minutes or until rankled on all sides, turning at times. Move to a medium bowl. In the mean time, in a little skillet heat oil over medium intensity. Add garlic and squashed red pepper; cook around 5 minutes or until garlic is brilliant, mixing every now and again.

Pour oil combination over broccoli, throwing to cover. Let stand 10 minutes. Mix in lemon strip, lemon squeeze and salt.

Tips

Tip: Ensure the broccoli is totally dry prior to cooking to keep it from steaming in the dish.

Day 7

- **Breakfast**: Beans on toast
- **Morning snack:** Turmeric latte

Cook Time:10 mins

Total Time:10 mins

Servings:1

Yield:1 serving

Ingredients

1 cup unsweetened almond milk or coconut milk drink

1 tablespoon ground new turmeric

2 teaspoons unadulterated maple syrup or honey

1 teaspoon ground new ginger

Touch of ground pepper

1 squeeze Ground cinnamon for embellish

Bearings

Consolidate milk, turmeric, maple syrup (or honey), ginger and pepper in a blender. Process on high until exceptionally smooth, around 1 moment. Fill a little pan and intensity over medium-high intensity until steaming hot yet not bubbling. Move to a mug. Embellish with a sprinkle of cinnamon, whenever wanted.

Lunch : Avocado egg salad sandwich

Prep Time:20 mins

Total Time:20 mins

Servings:2

Yield:2 sandwiches

Ingredients

½ ready avocado

1 ½ teaspoons lemon juice

1 teaspoon avocado oil

3 hard-bubbled eggs, cleaved

¼ cup finely cleaved celery (around 1 stem)

1 tablespoon cut new chives

¼ teaspoon salt

⅛ teaspoon ground pepper

4 cuts entire wheat sandwich bread, toasted

2 leaves lettuce

Bearings

Scoop the tissue from the avocado half into a medium bowl. Add lemon squeeze and oil; squash until generally smooth. Add slashed eggs, celery, chives, salt and pepper and mix to join. Split the combination between 2 cuts of toast. Top each with a piece of lettuce and one more cut of toast.

- **Dinner**: One pot garlicky shrimp & spinach

Active Time:25 mins

Total Time:25 mins

Servings:4

Yield:4 cups

Ingredient

3 tablespoons extra-virgin olive oil, isolated

6 medium cloves garlic, cut, isolated

1 pound spinach

¼ teaspoon salt in addition to 1/8 teaspoon, isolated

1 tablespoon lemon juice

1 pound shrimp (21-30 count), stripped and deveined

¼ teaspoon squashed red pepper

1 tablespoon finely cleaved new parsley

1 ½ teaspoons lemon zing

Bearings

Heat 1 tablespoon oil in a huge pot over medium intensity. Add a portion of the garlic and cook until starting to brown, 1 to 2 minutes. Add spinach and 1/4 teaspoon salt and throw to cover. Cook, mixing on more than one occasion, until for the most part withered, 3 to 5 minutes. Eliminate from intensity and mix in lemon juice. Transfer to a bowl, then keep heated.

Increment intensity to medium-high and add the excess 2 tablespoons of oil to the pot. Add the leftover garlic and cook until starting to brown, 1 to 2 minutes. Add shrimp, crushed red pepper and the excess 1/8 teaspoon salt; cook, blending, until the shrimp are simply cooked through, 3 to 5 minutes more. Serve the shrimp over the spinach, sprinkled with lemon zing and parsley.

Chapter 8: Conclusion

As you journey through the pages of "Simple Healing," you've embarked on a transformative exploration of anti-inflammatory eating, paving the way for enhanced well-being and vitality. As we conclude this culinary adventure, it's essential to equip you with the tools and resources to seamlessly integrate these principles into your daily life.

Planning an Anti-Inflammatory Week:

Harness the power of proactive planning by crafting a weekly menu that embraces anti-inflammatory ingredients and flavors. Consider incorporating a balance of vibrant fruits, vegetables, lean proteins, and healthy fats, ensuring a diverse array of nutrients and culinary experiences. By dedicating time to plan your meals, you foster consistency, creativity, and commitment to your wellness journey.

Grocery Shopping Guide:

Navigate the aisles with confidence using our comprehensive Grocery Shopping Guide. Familiarize yourself with essential anti-inflammatory staples, from nutrient-rich leafy greens and colorful berries to omega-3-packed fish and wholesome grains. Prioritize organic, locally sourced options when feasible, and remember to stock up on pantry staples that facilitate effortless meal preparation and enjoyment.

Storage and Reheating Tips:
Maximize freshness and flavor retention with our expert Storage and Reheating Tips. Invest in quality storage containers, practice proper food storage techniques, and utilize refrigerator and freezer-friendly options to extend shelf life without compromising nutritional integrity. Embrace mindful reheating practices, ensuring even heat distribution and preserving the texture and taste of your culinary creations.

Additional Resources and Reading:
Continue your exploration of anti-inflammatory living with our curated selection of Additional Resources and Reading. Delve deeper into the science of nutrition, explore holistic health practices, and discover inspiring literature that reinforces your commitment to vibrant health and well-being. Whether you're seeking recipe inspiration, nutritional insights, or motivational guidance, these resources serve as invaluable companions on your journey.

In essence, "Simple Healing" transcends the confines of a traditional cookbook; it's a holistic guide, empowering you to embrace a nourishing, anti-inflammatory lifestyle with confidence, creativity, and conviction. By integrating these principles into your daily life and leveraging the tools and resources provided, you cultivate a foundation for sustained health, happiness, and harmony for years to come. Embrace the journey, savor each moment, and celebrate the transformative power of nourishing, anti-inflammatory living.

Following "Simple Healing" Step-by-Step

Embarking on the "Simple Healing" journey necessitates a thoughtful, step-by-step approach to ensure you derive the maximum benefits from this transformative cookbook.

Introduction & Understanding: Begin by immersing yourself in the introductory sections, acquainting yourself with the fundamentals of inflammation, the benefits of an anti-inflammatory diet, and key nutrients that combat inflammation. Understanding the underlying principles sets the stage for a meaningful culinary experience.

Recipe Selection: Browse through the diverse array of recipes, from energizing breakfast options to satisfying dinners and delectable desserts. Prioritize recipes that resonate with your tastes, dietary preferences, and nutritional goals, ensuring a personalized and enjoyable experience.

Meal Planning: Dedicate time to craft a weekly meal plan, incorporating a variety of recipes to foster culinary diversity and nutrient balance. Tailor your selections based on seasonal availability, dietary requirements, and lifestyle considerations, ensuring practicality and sustainability.

Grocery Shopping: Utilize the comprehensive Grocery Shopping Guide to procure high-quality ingredients that align with the anti-inflammatory principles outlined in the cookbook. Prioritize organic, locally sourced options whenever possible, fostering a connection with your food and supporting sustainable practices.

Preparation & Cooking: Embrace the joy of cooking as you navigate each recipe, following the step-by-step instructions meticulously. Emphasize mindful preparation techniques, savoring each ingredient's texture, aroma, and flavor. Incorporate love and intention into each dish, fostering a deeper connection with your culinary creations.

Storage & Reheating: Leverage the Storage and Reheating Tips to maintain optimal freshness, flavor, and nutritional integrity. Practice proper storage techniques, utilize quality containers, and embrace mindful reheating practices to preserve the essence of each recipe.

Reflect & Adapt: As you progress through the cookbook, reflect on your experiences, preferences, and feedback. Adapt recipes based on your evolving tastes, nutritional needs, and culinary creativity, fostering a dynamic and personalized approach to anti-inflammatory living.

Leave a Comment

Your feedback is invaluable, serving as a beacon of guidance, inspiration, and motivation for fellow readers and future editions of "Simple Healing." Please take a moment to share your thoughts, experiences, and insights, highlighting your favorite recipes, transformative moments, and suggestions for improvement. Your voice contributes to a vibrant community of health enthusiasts, fostering collaboration, growth, and collective well-being. Embrace this opportunity to connect, inspire, and celebrate the transformative power of nourishing, anti-inflammatory living.